Table of Contents

INTRODUCTION 3

CHAPTER ONE 4

WHAT IS SJÖGREN'S SYNDROME? 4

WHO MIGHT GET SJÖGREN'S SYNDROME? 4

SYMPTOMS AND CAUSES 5

DIAGNOSIS AND TESTS 6

MANAGEMENT AND TREATMENT 7

WHAT ARE THE COMPLICATIONS OF SJÖGREN'S SYNDROME? 12

PREVENTION 13

OUTLOOK / PROGNOSIS 13

NUTRITION AND SJÖGREN'S SYNDROME 17

FOODS TO AVOID 18

FOODS TO EAT 19

TOP 14 FOODS FOODS FOR A SJOGREN'S SYNDROME DIET . 20

CHAPTER TWO 27

Gluten-Free Casserole 27

Easy Gluten-Free Turkey Burgers 30

Kitchen Sink Soup 32

Turkey Frame Vegetable Soup 34

Bacon-Mushroom Turkey Burger 36

Vegetable Soup - Irish Style 38

Chocolate Chip Cookies for Special Diets 40
Gluten-Free Chocolate Chip Cookies 42
Guilt-Free Cream of Asparagus Soup 44
Grain Free and Gluten Free Chocolate Chip Cookies 47
Juicy Slow Cooker Chicken Breast for Any Diet 50
Lemon Garlic Chicken Breasts 51
Quick and Easy Chicken and Ham Corn Chowder 53
Balsamic Marinated Chicken Breasts 55
Sugar-Free Whole Wheat Pumpkin Bran Muffins with Raisins 57
Whole Wheat Pumpkin Coffee Cake Muffins 60
Homemade Wonderful Bread 62
Light Oat Bread 64
Marbled Chocolate-Pumpkin Muffins 65
CONCLUSIONS 70

INTRODUCTION

The Sjögren's syndrome diet is a food-based approach to reducing inflammation and other symptoms of Sjögren's syndrome. While not a cure for this autoimmune condition, modifying your diet can help to treat symptoms, provide a higher quality of life, and improve your overall health.

CHAPTER ONE

WHAT IS SJÖGREN'S SYNDROME?

Sjögren's syndrome is a lifelong autoimmune disorder that reduces the amount of moisture produced by glands in the eyes and mouth. It is named for Henrik Sjögren, a Swedish eye doctor who first described the condition. While dry mouth and dry eyes are the primary symptoms, most people who have these problems don't have Sjögren's syndrome. Dry mouth is also called xerostomia.

There are two forms of Sjögren's syndrome:

- Primary Sjögren's syndrome develops on its own, not because of any other health condition.
- Secondary Sjögren's syndrome develops in addition to other autoimmune diseases like rheumatoid arthritis, lupus and psoriatic arthritis.

WHO MIGHT GET SJÖGREN'S SYNDROME?

An estimated one to four million Americans have Sjögren's syndrome. The disease affects people of all races, ethnicities and ages. However, women are nine times more likely to develop this condition than men.

What causes Sjögren's syndrome?

Sjögren's syndrome is an autoimmune disease, which means something triggers your immune system to attack healthy cells. This attack damages the tear system in your eyes and the salivary glands in your mouth. Exactly what causes this abnormal immune system response is not clear. These factors may play a role:

- Environmental factors.
- Genetics.
- Sex hormones (the condition affects more women than men).
- Viral infections.

What are the symptoms of Sjögren's syndrome?

In addition to extremely dry eyes and mouth, some people experience muscle pain and joint pain all over the body, similar to fibromyalgia. Other symptoms include:

- Abnormal sense of taste.
- Burning or redness in eyes, or grittiness (like sand).
- Blurry vision.

- Difficulty chewing, swallowing or talking.
- Dry cough or hoarseness.
- Dry, itchy skin.
- Enlarged salivary glands.
- Fatigue.
- Tooth decay or early tooth loss.
- Vaginal dryness.

DIAGNOSIS AND TESTS

How is Sjögren's syndrome diagnosed?

If you have dry mouth, dry eyes or other signs of Sjögren's syndrome, your doctor may use these methods to confirm a diagnosis:

- Blood tests: These tests detect specific antibodies in the blood. They look for anti-nuclear antibodies (ANA), anti-Sjögren's syndrome antibodies (anti-SSA, also called anti-Ro) and anti-Sjögren's syndrome type B (anti-SSB, also called anti-La). A blood test can also detect rheumatoid factor, an antibody found in many people who have rheumatoid arthritis.

- Biopsy: Your doctor may remove tissue or cells from a salivary gland or the inside of your lip. This biopsy sample goes to a lab to check for signs of inflammation.
- Eye exam: An eye specialist, such as an ophthalmologist, can measure tear production. During an eye exam, your doctor will examine the cornea, the clear part of the eye, for dryness.
- Imaging tests: These include sialometry, which measures how much saliva you produce by using X-rays that can see dye injected into salivary glands. There is also salivary scintigraphy, a way to track how long it takes for a radioactive isotope to travel from an injection point in your vein to your salivary glands.
- Health history: If you have a pre-existing autoimmune disease, plus dry eyes and dry mouth, your doctor may conclude that you have developed secondary Sjögren's syndrome.

MANAGEMENT AND TREATMENT

What kind of a doctor treats Sjögren's syndrome?

Many types of doctors might be involved in your care if you have SS. These include your own primary care provider, your dentist, and specialists such as rheumatologists, ophthalmologists and otolaryngologists, also called ear, nose and throat (ENT) doctors.

How is Sjögren's syndrome managed or treated?

There is no cure for Sjögren's syndrome, but treatments can relieve symptoms. Depending on your specific issues, your doctor may recommend one or more of these therapies.

Treatments for dry eyes:

- Artificial tears: Over-the-counter artificial tear eye solutions and artificial tear eye ointments moisturize dry eyes. These products relieve irritation and discomfort.
- Prescription eye drops: Cyclosporine and lifitegrast prescription eye drops soothe inflamed tear glands and stimulate tear production.
- Punctal plugs: An ophthalmologist inserts tiny silicone plugs into the tear ducts. The plugs block the ducts so tears stay on the eyes, keeping them wet.

- Surgery: If punctal plugs work for you, your doctor may recommend surgery to close the tear ducts permanently.
- Autologous serum drops: Your doctor can make customized artificial tears. The process involves mixing your blood serum (a clear liquid separated from your blood) with a sterile liquid solution. You receive a one-of-a-kind tear substitute unique to your body. While effective, the pricey treatment isn't always covered by insurance.
- Treatments for dry mouth:

- Saliva producers: Products such as gum and hard candies that contain sweeteners like sorbitol or xylitol can stimulate saliva production. You can also use an over-the-counter or prescription saliva substitute. Prescription products include sorbitol oral lozenges and sorbitol oromucosal solutions (solutions that are directed toward the cheeks).

- Prescription medications: Pilocarpine (Salagen®) and cevimeline (Evoxac®) pills increase the natural production of saliva.
- Dental care: A dry mouth increases the risk of dental cavities, infections and tooth decay. Your doctor may recommend a prescription toothpaste and mouthwash, as well as regular fluoride treatments.
- Treatments for joint or organ problems:

- Over-the-counter pain relievers: Acetaminophen (Tylenol®) and nonsteroidal anti-inflammatory drugs (NSAIDs), such as ibuprofen (Motrin®) and naproxen (Aleve®), can relieve joint pain and muscle aches.
- Anti-rheumatics: Hydroxychloroquine prescription pills can diminish pain from rheumatoid arthritis or lupus. This medication may also reduce salivary gland swelling.
- Immunosuppressants: These prescription medications slow the immune system's response.

They lessen inflammation and prevent organ damage.

- Steroids: Prednisone prescription pills soothe inflammation of the joints, skin and organs.
- Antifungals: These medications treat yeast overgrowth in your mouth (oral thrush) or in your vagina (vaginal yeast infection).
- Treatments for vaginal dryness:

If your vagina is always dry, itchy and sore, you should check with your healthcare provider to make sure that the issue is not something more than hormonal changes. You might have some type of infection or skin issue. These conditions would require specific treatments. In general, though, women with Sjögren's syndrome are two to three times more likely to have issues with vaginal dryness and atrophy than women of similar ages around and after menopause. Tips for helping with everyday vaginal dryness include:

Trying vaginal moisturizers or lubricants to add moisture to the vagina daily and to ease sexual intercourse.

Using unscented soaps for cleansing. Perfumes and other additives can cause irritation.

Asking your healthcare provider about vaginal estrogen therapy.

WHAT ARE THE COMPLICATIONS OF SJÖGREN'S SYNDROME?

Most people who have Sjögren's syndrome live their lives without any significant problems. However, a dry mouth means that you are more likely to have dental problems, such as tooth decay and infection. Dry eyes can also place you at risk for eye infections.

If you have secondary Sjögren's syndrome, you may also have problems like joint paint caused by rheumatoid arthritis or lupus. Rarely, people with Sjögren's syndrome develop these complications:

- Abnormal liver or kidney function.
- Lymphomas (cancerous tumors in the lymph nodes).
- Lung problems that may be mistaken for pneumonia.
- Neurological problems that cause weakness or numbness.
- Skin rashes (red skin).

PREVENTION

How can I prevent Sjögren's syndrome?

Because no one knows exactly what causes Sjögren's syndrome or other autoimmune diseases, there is no known way to prevent it.

OUTLOOK / PROGNOSIS

What is the prognosis (outlook) for people with Sjögren's syndrome?

Constantly having a dry mouth or dry eyes is certainly uncomfortable. Fortunately, symptoms tend to lessen over time. With the right therapies, you can manage symptoms so they do not interfere with your ability to enjoy life.

Does Sjögren's syndrome cause weight gain?

Sjögren's syndrome doesn't cause weight gain. However, medications (like steroids) used to treat symptoms may cause weight gain. Also, there are conditions like hypothyroidism that may be linked to Sjögren's syndrome that can result in unintended weight gain.

Does Sjögren's syndrome affect ears?

Sjögren's syndrome, like other autoimmune conditions, can affect ears, too. You might have trouble with hearing loss or with balance.

What should I eat if I have Sjögren's syndrome? What foods should I avoid?

An estimated 90% of people with Sjögren's syndrome have problems related to eating. In some cases, these problems can be enough to cause malnutrition. Troubles can be related to dryness and swelling of the throat, as well as intestinal tract or nerve damage. There also seems to be a significant number of people who have both Sjögren's syndrome and celiac disease and/or symptoms of irritable bowel syndrome (bloating, abdominal pain, diarrhea and/or constipation).

If you have gastrointestinal symptoms, you can work with a registered dietitian (RD) to find out what food sensitivities you have. An RD can then also help you to create a food plan that works well for you and provides the nutrients you need.

Problems with gastroesophageal reflux (GERD) are also common among people in general and among people with Sjögren's syndrome in particular. Your care team can provide you with tips for dealing with GERD. These might include not eating two to three hours before you lie down to sleep and avoiding greasy foods. There are some recommendations that people who have autoimmune disorders like Sjögren's syndrome should follow an anti-inflammatory diet to help with joint pain and other symptoms. Some people have found relief from a completely plant-based diet.

Here are some tips that might help you manage other types of eating issues:

Eat smaller amounts of food at one time, but eat more frequently throughout the day.

Include soft foods in your diet.

Be sure to chew your food completely.

Avoid cavities by reducing the amount of sugar you eat and drinking only water before you go to bed.

Is Sjögren's syndrome considered a disability?

The U.S. government has awarded disability to people with severe cases of Sjögren's syndrome. However, this is a question that you should discuss with your healthcare provider to see if you are eligible.

Does Sjögren's syndrome cause hair loss?

If you have Sjögren's syndrome, you might see some hair loss, and it might be as a result of the condition. There is a condition known as frontal fibrosing alopecia that is being found in higher numbers in people (mostly women) with autoimmune diseases. This condition causes slow hair loss at the front hairline and sometimes the eyebrows.

However, hair loss can be triggered by many things, including stressful life events and medications. You should ask your dermatologist about problems with hair loss.

When should I call the doctor if I have Sjögren's syndrome?

Severe mouth or gum pain could indicate infection or tooth decay. Itchy eyes, eye pain, or blurred or double vision can signal infections or other vision problems. You should also call your doctor if you notice swollen lymph nodes in your neck, armpits or groin. Enlarged lymph nodes could indicate lymphoma or another health condition.

What questions should I ask my doctor if I have Sjögren's syndrome?

If you have Sjögren's syndrome, you may want to ask your doctor:

What lifestyle measures can I take to make my symptoms more livable?

Can certain medications, drinks or foods dry out the eyes or mouth?

Should I look out for any signs of complications?

While there isn't a cure for the dry mouth, dry eyes or other problems caused by Sjögren's syndrome, you don't have to live with discomfort or pain. Talk openly with your healthcare provider about how the disease affects your everyday life. Eating, swallowing, speaking and seeing are all critical for enjoying life. Your provider can help you find the right combination of therapies to relieve symptoms.

NUTRITION AND SJÖGREN'S SYNDROME

Similar to many recommended diets, the Sjögren's syndrome diet focuses on well-balanced meals rich with vegetables, lean proteins, and fruits. Other than increasing nutrients and healthy proteins in your diet, the Sjögren's diet reduces or eliminates foods that can cause inflammation or trigger allergic reactions.

Combined with a prescribed treatment plan, a moderated diet can help to prevent or reduce dryness and inflammation from Sjögren's syndrome.

FOODS TO AVOID

Pursuing the Sjögren's diet or a similar anti-inflammatory diet means eliminating common trigger foods and allergens.

Some foods to avoid include:

- red meat
- processed foods
- fried foods
- dairy
- sugars and sweets
- alcohol
- soda
- gluten
- refined grains
- safflower, corn, and canola oils

Some foods affect people differently. Though these foods can trigger inflammation and worsen Sjögren's syndrome symptoms, some can be eaten in moderation. This specifically applies to some dairy products, such as yogurt and cheese.

If your symptoms begin to worsen after eating specific foods, consider eliminating them from your diet. Also, discuss your symptoms with your doctor to ensure you receive the best treatment.

FOODS TO EAT

Maintaining a diet rich in foods with anti-inflammatory effects can reduce dryness symptoms and provide relief from other associated conditions. Some foods high in anti-inflammatory benefits include:

- leafy green vegetables
- nuts
- fruits
- turmeric
- ginger
- garlic
- fatty fish
- olives and olive oil
- avocado
- whole grains

How you cook your foods can also affect dry mouth symptoms. Here are some additional tips to make your meals more enjoyable:

If you choose to make a sandwich, consider adding vegetables that are high in moisture, such as cucumbers.

Adding sauces to your meals can ease swallowing, but use creamy sauces in moderation to limit fat content.

Try soups and smoothies as alternatives to dry foods.

Drink with your meals to ease swallowing.

Soften your foods with broth.

Tender-cook your meats to prevent them from drying out

TOP 14 FOODS FOODS FOR A SJOGREN'S SYNDROME DIET

When the immune system attacks real or imagined threats, inflammation is a result. This sequence brings about pain, swelling, and redness in the affected area. Any part of the body can be a target: skin, joints, muscles, nerves, and internal organs.

Medications like Plaquenil and methotrexate have a positive effect on immune system response. However, a Sjogren's syndrome diet, by stressing foods that reduce inflammation, is on the front lines in the battle against this (and any) autoimmune disease. These foods are vital soldiers in the campaign to quiet a haywire immune system.

1. Healthy Fats

While many fatty foodstuffs, including margarine and canola and corn oils, are off-limits because they can set off inflammation, there are healthy fats that should be part of a Sjogren's syndrome diet. Olive oil (especially the extra virgin type) is high in omega 3 fatty acids. Other helpful foods are salmon, tuna, sardines, mackerel, avocados, nuts, and some kinds of seeds.

2. Vegetables

The brighter the color, the more important nutrients veggies contain. Carrots, green beans, sweet potatoes, and winter squash are delicious sources of protective vitamin A and vitamin C. Produce is better eaten raw and unpeeled, as valuable nutrients are lost to cooking and peeling.

3. Fruit

The same goes for fruit. Try blueberries, apples, honeydew melon, and papaya by themselves or added to yogurt for a tasty, inflammation-blasting addition to your daily fare.

4. Fiber

People with Sjogren's syndrome can have more than dry eyes and mouth. The digestive system also may feel the effects of too little moisture. Fiber can help the intestines move. Flax seeds and quinoa (pronounced keen-wah) work wonders.

5. Liquids

Liquids are an all-important part of a Sjogren's syndrome diet. Drinks of all kinds (preferably without added sugar) should be a part of the food regimen. Juice, seltzer, and herbal teas add variety. Coconut water is an increasingly popular beverage with an added benefit: it is high in energy-boosting potassium that can jump-start a worn-out Sjogren patient's day.

6. Moist Foods

Foods containing healthy amounts of moisture like sauces, mayonnaise, and yogurt can keep dryness at bay. Soup and stew have a double advantage: they not only add much-needed liquid to the diet but contain vegetables and other helpful ingredients.

7. Organic Meat

Red meat can increase inflammation, but there is one exception. Cows and bison that eat grass rather than livestock feed are good sources of anti-inflammatory fats. Free-range chicken and eggs are also beneficial additions to a Sjogren's syndrome diet. Be sure to prepare them in a Sjogren's-friendly manner. Steaming and cooking in a liquid is much better than broiling or frying.

8. Protein

The sky is the limit for this important part of a Sjogren's syndrome diet. Think beyond meat, poultry, and eggs. Lentils, chickpeas (aka garbanzo beans), peas, and nut butter are all good sources of protein.

9. Whole Grains

Buckwheat, wild and brown rice, quinoa, millet, and amaranth are chock-full of important nutrients. In addition, since they are cooked in water, these grains are high in liquid—a boon for people living with dry eyes, mouths, and nasal passages.

10. Nuts and Seeds

Almonds, pistachios, walnuts, and cashews are good sources of protein, calcium, and other necessary nutrients. And along with sesame, chia, and other seeds, they provide an all-important fiber boost.

11. Herbs and Spices

Don't forget the seasoning. These flavor enhancers are an important addition to a Sjogren's syndrome diet. Ginger, garlic, and turmeric are anti-inflammatory. Carob powder, parsley (a source of vitamin C), and dill add to the flavor of many foods. For an extra bonus, use ginger on salmon, chicken, and winter squash for a delicious and healthful dish.

12. Easily-Digested Foods

A Sjogren's syndrome diet should consist of foods that go down easily. Since the digestive system from top to bottom may be irritated by a lack of moisture, this fare can make sure people can eat properly without discomfort. Soft vegetables, low-acid fruit, tender cuts of meat and chicken (not broiled or fried), and grains are definitely on the menu.

13. Gluten-Free Foods

Sjogren's syndrome and gluten sensitivity go hand-in-hand. According to studies, as many as 14.7% of people with the disorder have celiac disease. And nearly half of Sjogren's patients cannot tolerate gluten. With numbers like these, it makes sense to eliminate this protein—found in wheat, rye, and other grains—from the diet. Instead, fill up on rice, vegetables, fruit, legumes, eggs, fish, chicken, and turkey. (One patient also saw a marked improvement when she stopped eating dairy.)

Leafy Greens (and Reds)

The Sjogren's syndrome diet would not be complete without these nutritional powerhouses. Kale, spinach, red and green leaf lettuce, broccoli, romaine lettuce, and their cousins are outstanding sources of vitamins A, C, and K. Several leafy vegetables boast beneficial levels of folate, calcium, and folate. Even though some—like collards and mustard greens—are cooked, many can be eaten raw. There's only one drawback: Swiss chard and spinach contain oxalates, which can cause kidney stones. Cooking reduces this risk.

14. Alternate Milk

Many people with Sjogren's have difficulty with dairy, but this does not mean they have to give up their morning cereal or latte. Milk made from rice, almonds, cashews, and coconut is a tasty substitute. These alternative milk products either naturally contain or are fortified with essential nutrients.

CHAPTER TWO

Gluten-Free Casserole

Recipe Summary

Prep: 25 mins

Cook: 45 mins

Additional: 10 mins

Total: 1 hr 20 mins

Servings: 8

Yield: 8 servings

Ingredients

- 8 cups water
- 2 cups green beans, chopped
- 1 teaspoon extra-virgin olive oil
- 1 small onion, chopped fine
- 1 ½ pounds ground turkey
- salt and ground black pepper to taste
- 5 cloves garlic, minced
- 2 tablespoons chopped fresh basil
- 2 teaspoons chopped fresh thyme

- 1 cup frozen peas
- 1 cup mushrooms, chopped
- 2 zucchini, chopped
- 2 cups crushed tomatoes
- 1 cup shredded mozzarella cheese
- 2 tablespoons freshly grated Parmesan cheese

Directions

Step 1

Bring water to a boil in a large pot. Cook green beans at a boil until just softened, about 3 minutes; drain.

Step 2

Preheat oven to 350 degrees F (175 degrees C).

Step 3

Heat olive oil in a large skillet over medium-low heat. Cook and stir onion in hot oil until translucent, 3 to 5 minutes.

Step 4

Crumble ground turkey into the skillet and increase heat to medium-high. Season turkey generously with salt and pepper; cook and stir until the turkey is completely browned,

7 to 10 minutes. Reduce heat to medium. Stir garlic, basil, and thyme through the turkey mixture; cook, stirring occasionally, another 3 minutes.

Step 5

Remove turkey mixture from skillet with a slotted spoon and transfer to a 9x13-inch casserole dish. Reserve 2 tablespoons of the pan drippings for later use and discard remainder.

Step 6

Heat the reserved pan drippings in the skillet over medium heat. Stir green beans, peas, mushrooms, and zucchini into the hot pan drippings; season with salt and black pepper. Cook and stir vegetable mixture until hot, about 5 minutes; add to casserole dish and stir to combine. Pour crushed tomatoes over the turkey and vegetable mixture. Top with a layer of mozzarella cheese. Sprinkle Parmesan cheese over the mozzarella cheese.

Step 7

Bake in preheated oven until the cheese is melted and vegetables are tender, about 20 minutes. Rest dish 10 minutes before serving.

Nutrition Facts

Per Serving: 217 calories; protein 23.6g; carbohydrates 9.6g; fat 9.9g; cholesterol 73mg; sodium 191mg.

Easy Gluten-Free Turkey Burgers

Recipe Summary

Prep: 5 mins

Cook: 14 mins

Total: 19 mins

Servings: 5

Yield: 5 burgers

Ingredients

- 1 pound ground turkey
- ½ white onion, finely chopped
- ¼ cup almond flour
- 1 large egg
- 3 cloves garlic, minced
- 2 sprigs fresh basil, chopped
- 1 pinch garlic and herb seasoning blend (such as Mrs. Dash®), or to taste

- ground black pepper to taste

Directions

Step 1

Preheat grill for medium heat and lightly oil the grate.

Step 2

Mix ground turkey, onion, almond flour, egg, garlic, basil, seasoning blend, and black pepper together thoroughly in a bowl. Form 5 burger patties using about 1/3 cup of the turkey mixture for each.

Step 3

Cook turkey burgers on preheated grill until no longer pink in the center and the juices run clear, 7 to 10 minutes per side. An instant-read thermometer inserted into the center should read at least 165 degrees F (74 degrees C).

Cook's Notes:

The seasoning I used is a Mrs. Dash(R) blend. You can substitute it for seasonings like garlic powder, parsley, oregano, thyme, coriander, cayenne pepper, cumin, or rosemary to make your own.

A burger press comes in handy for forming the burger patties.

Nutrition Facts

Per Serving: 192 calories; protein 20.8g; carbohydrates 3.2g; fat 10.9g; cholesterol 104.1mg; sodium 66.1mg.

Kitchen Sink Soup

Recipe Summary

Prep: 20 mins

Cook: 30 mins

Total: 50 mins

Servings: 10

Yield: 10 servings

Ingredients

- 10 cups chicken broth
- 2 potatoes, cubed
- 2 carrots, sliced
- 2 stalks celery, diced
- 5 fresh mushrooms, sliced
- 1 green bell pepper, chopped

- 1 fresh broccoli, chopped
- 4 cups cauliflower florets
- 1 parsnip, sliced
- 1 onion, chopped
- 1 cup green peas
- 1 cup cut green beans, drained
- 1 cup wax beans, drained
- ½ cup cooked chickpeas
- ½ cup cooked navy beans
- salt and pepper to taste
- 1 teaspoon dried parsley

Directions

Step 1

In a large stockpot, combine all the ingredients and cook over medium heat partially covered for about 30 minutes or until all the vegetables are tender. Serve hot with buttered biscuits.

Nutrition Facts

Per Serving: 160 calories; protein 10.3g; carbohydrates 26.3g; fat 1.9g; sodium 1008.1mg.

Turkey Frame Vegetable Soup

Recipe Summary

Prep: 1 hr 30 mins

Cook: 1 hr 20 mins

Additional: 8 hrs

Total: 10 hrs 50 mins

Servings: 8

Yield: 8 servings

Ingredients

- 1 turkey carcass
- 2 carrots, chopped
- 2 stalks celery, cut into 2 inch pieces
- 1 onions, chopped
- 4 cloves garlic, minced
- 4 sprigs fresh parsley
- 12 black peppercorns
- 2 bay leaves
- 1 teaspoon dried thyme
- 1 tablespoon chicken bouillon granules

- 8 cups water
- water to cover
- 1 turnip, peeled and cubed
- 2 parsnips, peeled and sliced
- 3 carrots, chopped
- ½ cup frozen green beans
- ½ cup frozen green peas
- 1 (15 ounce) can red beans, drained and rinsed
- ¼ cup chopped fresh parsley

Directions

Step 1

Place turkey carcass in a large pot over high heat. Add the carrots, celery, onion, garlic, parsley sprigs, peppercorns, bay leaves, thyme, chicken bouillon granules, water and enough water to cover all. Bring to a boil, uncovered, then reduce heat to medium low and let simmer for 1 1/2 hours.

Step 2

Remove the turkey carcass and allow it to cool. Remove any meat from the carcass, cut into bite-sized pieces and set aside. Strain the stock through a sieve OR a colander covered with cheesecloth into another large pot. Discard the unstrained ingredients. Place the turkey meat into the pot, cover and refrigerate overnight.

Step 3

The next day, use a slotted spoon to remove the fat that has solidified on top of the stock. Return the stock to a large pot over high heat, add the turnip, parsnips and carrots and bring to a boil. Reduce heat to low, cover and simmer for one hour, or until vegetables are tender.

Step 4

Add the green beans, peas and beans and allow to heat through, about 15 minutes. Finally add the chopped parsley and season with salt and pepper to taste.

Nutrition Facts

Per Serving: 133 calories; protein 5.7g; carbohydrates 25.1g; fat 2g; cholesterol 3.8mg; sodium 314.2mg.

Bacon-Mushroom Turkey Burger

Recipe Summary

Prep: 15 mins

Cook: 12 mins

Total: 27 mins

Servings: 4

Yield: 4 burgers

Ingredients

- 2 slices multigrain bread
- 1 pound ground turkey
- 6 white mushrooms, finely chopped
- 1 egg
- 2 green onions, finely chopped
- 3 slices cooked bacon, finely chopped, or more to taste
- 5 dashes hot sauce, or more to taste
- ½ teaspoon pureed garlic
- salt and ground black pepper to taste

Directions

Step 1

Mince bread in a food processor and transfer crumbs to a bowl. Add turkey, mushrooms, egg, green onions, bacon, hot sauce, garlic, salt, and pepper. Mix well and divide into 4 portions. Form each portion into a patty.

Step 2

Preheat a grill for medium heat and lightly oil the grate. Cook patties until no longer pink in the center, 12 to 14 minutes.

Cook's Notes:

You can substitute panko bread crumbs for the crumbled bread, or use sprouted grain bread. End pieces are preferable.

You can mince the mushrooms in the food processor.

Use turkey bacon, if you prefer.

You can replace the chopped bacon with 1/3 cup bacon bits.

Nutrition Facts

Per Serving: 228 calories; protein 26.7g; carbohydrates 7.3g; fat 10.4g; cholesterol 130.1mg; sodium 210.5mg.

Vegetable Soup - Irish Style

Recipe Summary

Prep: 10 mins

Cook: 20 mins

Total: 30 mins

Servings: 6

Yield: 6 servings

Ingredients

- 3 carrots, chopped
- 3 large potatoes - peeled and cubed
- 1 parsnip, peeled and diced
- 1 turnip, peeled and diced
- 1 leek, sliced
- ½ onion, chopped
- ¼ cup dry potato flakes (Optional)
- salt and pepper to taste
- 1 cup water, or as needed

Directions

Step 1

Place the carrots, potatoes, parsnip, turnip, leek and onion into a large saucepan. Fill with enough water to cover. Bring to a boil and cook until the vegetables are tender. Drain off water and puree vegetables in a blender or using a stick blender.

Step 2

Return the puree to the saucepan and stir in water to reach your desired thickness. Heat to a simmer and season with salt and pepper. Serve and enjoy.

Nutrition Facts

Per Serving: 198 calories; protein 5g; carbohydrates 45.2g; fat 0.4g; sodium 53.5mg.

Chocolate Chip Cookies for Special Diets

Recipe Summary

Prep: 15 mins

Cook: 12 mins

Additional: 23 mins

Total: 50 mins

Servings: 48

Yield: 4 dozen

Ingredients

- ½ cup butter, softened
- ¾ cup granulated artificial sweetener
- 2 tablespoons water
- ½ teaspoon vanilla extract
- 1 egg, beaten
- 1 ⅛ cups all-purpose flour
- ½ teaspoon baking soda
- ½ teaspoon salt
- ½ cup semisweet chocolate chips
- ½ cup chopped pecans

Directions

Step 1

Preheat oven to 375 degrees F (190 degrees C).

Step 2

In a medium bowl, cream together the butter and sugar substitute. Mix in water, vanilla, and egg. Sift together the flour, baking soda, and salt; stir into the creamed mixture. Mix in the chocolate chips and pecans. Drop cookies by heaping teaspoonfuls onto a cookie sheet.

Step 3

Bake in the preheated oven for 10 to 12 minutes. Remove from cookie sheets to cool on wire racks. These cookies freeze well.

Nutrition Facts

Per Serving: 60 calories; protein 4.2g; carbohydrates 3.5g; fat 3.4g; cholesterol 9mg; sodium 53.8mg.

Gluten-Free Chocolate Chip Cookies

Recipe Summary

Prep: 15 mins

Cook: 10 mins

Additional: 10 mins

Total: 35 mins

Servings: 24

Yield: 2 dozen

Ingredients

- ½ cup coconut palm sugar
- ¼ cup extra-virgin coconut oil, at room temperature
- ½ teaspoon baking soda

- Himalayan pink salt to taste
- 2 cups almond flour
- 2 eggs
- 1 tablespoon vanilla extract
- 1 cup chocolate chips (such as Ghirardelli®)

Directions

Step 1

Preheat oven to 350 degrees F (175 degrees C). Lightly grease a baking sheet.

Step 2

Combine coconut sugar, coconut oil, baking soda, and salt in a large bowl; beat with a handheld electric mixer until smooth. Add almond flour, eggs, and vanilla extract. Beat dough at medium speed, scraping the bottom and sides of the bowl, until well mixed, about 1 minute.

Step 3

Fold chocolate chips into the dough. Grease your palms lightly with coconut oil; drop tablespoonfuls of dough onto the baking sheet.

Step 4

Bake in the preheated oven until golden brown, 10 to 12 minutes. Let cool on the baking sheet, about 10 minutes.

Nutrition Facts

Per Serving: 139 calories; protein 3g; carbohydrates 11.2g; fat 9.9g; cholesterol 15.5mg; sodium 36.2mg.

Guilt-Free Cream of Asparagus Soup

Recipe Summary

Prep: 15 mins

Cook: 40 mins

Total: 55 mins

Servings: 6

Yield: 6 servings

Ingredients

- 2 small boiling potatoes
- ¼ cup fat-free sour cream
- 1 pound asparagus
- 6 cups vegetable broth

- 2 tablespoons olive oil
- 1 cup chopped onion
- 2 cloves garlic, crushed
- 1 (8 ounce) package sliced fresh mushrooms
- 1 clove garlic, crushed
- ¼ cup dry white wine (Optional)
- 1 pinch cayenne pepper
- salt and ground black pepper to taste

Directions

Step 1

Place the potatoes into a small pot with enough water to cover; bring to a boil, then reduce heat to medium-low, place a cover on the pot, and simmer until tender, about 20 minutes.

Step 2

Drain the potatoes and transfer to a bowl; add the sour cream and mash lightly; scrape into the bowl of a blender.

Step 3

Cut asparagus into 3 parts: woody ends, tips, and center pieces.

Step 4

Combine the woody ends of the asparagus with the vegetable broth in a stockpot; bring to a boil and cook until the woody ends are tender. Remove woody ends with a slotted spoon and discard.

Step 5

Remove 2 tablespoons broth to a bowl with the asparagus tips. Transfer remainder of stock to blender with the potatoes.

Step 6

Chop the middle segments of the asparagus.

Step 7

Heat olive oil in a skillet over low-heat; cook and stir the chopped asparagus, chopped onion, and 2 crushed cloves garlic in the hot oil until the asparagus is tender, about 10 minutes. Add to the broth in the blender, reserving oil in the skillet.

Step 8

Blend the mixture in the blender on high until smooth and creamy; return to the stockpot.

Cook and stir the sliced mushrooms and 1 crushed garlic clove in the remaining oil over medium-low heat until the mushrooms soften, 3 to 5 minutes. Add the white wine; cook another 1 to 2 minutes. Stir the mushroom mixture into the soup.

Step 10

Heat the asparagus tips and broth in the microwave for 2 minutes; stir into the soup.

Step 11

Season the soup with cayenne pepper, salt, and black pepper.

Nutrition Facts

Per Serving: 167 calories; protein 6g; carbohydrates 23.7g; fat 5.3g; cholesterol 1.7mg; sodium 485.3mg.

Grain Free and Gluten Free Chocolate Chip Cookies

Recipe Summary

Prep: 10 mins

Cook: 10 mins

Total: 20 mins

Servings: 40

Yield: 40 cookies

Ingredients

- 1 cup butter, at room temperature
- 1 cup packed light brown sugar
- 2 eggs, at room temperature
- 1 tablespoon vanilla extract
- 3 cups blanched almond flour
- ¼ cup coconut flour
- 1 ¼ teaspoons kosher salt
- 1 teaspoon baking soda
- 2 cups chocolate chips

Directions

Step 1

Preheat oven to 350 degrees F (175 degrees C). Line a baking sheet with parchment paper.

Step 2

Beat butter and brown sugar together in a bowl using an electric mixer or in a food processor until smooth and creamy. Mix eggs and vanilla extract into creamed butter mixture. Add almond flour, coconut flour, salt, and baking soda to creamed butter mixture and stir until dough is well mixed; fold in chocolate chips. Drop dough by the rounded teaspoon onto the prepared baking sheet.

Step 3

Bake in the preheated oven until edges of cookies are browned, 8 to 12 minutes.

Cook's Notes:

If you can't do dairy, change out the butter for the same amount of fat of your choice (palm shortening or what-have-you).

Feel free to mix in chopped walnuts if you like those in your cookies. Another variation would be white chocolate chips, macadamia and Craisins(R), etc.

Nutrition Facts

Per Serving: 141 calories; protein 4.1g; carbohydrates 13.2g; fat 8.9g; cholesterol 21.5mg; sodium 130.7mg.

Recipe Summary

Prep: 10 mins

Cook: 6 hrs

Total: 6 hrs 10 mins

Servings: 4

Yield: 4 servings

Ingredients

- 1 pound skinless, boneless chicken breast halves
- 1 (14.5 ounce) can petite diced tomatoes
- ¼ onion, chopped (Optional)
- 1 teaspoon Italian seasoning (Optional)
- 1 clove garlic, minced (Optional)

Directions

Step 1

Arrange chicken in a slow cooker. Pour tomatoes over chicken; add onion, Italian seasoning, and garlic.

Step 2

Cook on Low for 6 to 8 hours.

Cook's Note:

You can use any type of herb in place of the Italian seasoning.

Nutrition Facts

Per Serving: 144 calories; protein 23.1g; carbohydrates 5.2g; fat 2.4g; cholesterol 58.5mg; sodium 208mg.

Lemon Garlic Chicken Breasts

Recipe Summary

Prep: 10 mins

Cook: 25 mins

Total: 35 mins

Servings: 4

Yield: 4 servings

Ingredients

- cooking spray
- 1 clove garlic, minced
- 4 skinless, boneless chicken breast halves

- salt and ground black pepper to taste
- ¾ cup chicken broth
- 1 tablespoon lemon juice

Directions

Step 1

Lightly spray a nonstick skillet with cooking spray and place over low heat; cook and stir garlic until fragrant and lightly browned, 2 to 3 minutes.

Step 2

Season chicken with salt and pepper and place in skillet with garlic; cook over medium heat until browned on both sides, 10 to 12 minutes. Add chicken broth and lemon juice; bring to a boil. Reduce heat to medium-low, cover skillet, and simmer until chicken is no longer pink in the center, 10 to 15 minutes. An instant-read thermometer inserted into the center should read at least 165 degrees F (74 degrees C).

Step 3

Transfer chicken to a serving dish, reserving liquid in skillet. Continue simmering liquid until slightly reduced, about 3 minutes. Pour liquid over chicken.

Nutrition Facts

Per Serving: 131 calories; protein 23.8g; carbohydrates 0.8g; fat 2.9g; cholesterol 65.5mg; sodium 275.2mg.

Quick and Easy Chicken and Ham Corn Chowder

Recipe Summary

Prep: 15 mins

Cook: 20 mins

Total: 35 mins

Servings: 6

Yield: 6 servings

Ingredients

- 1 tablespoon bacon drippings
- 1 cup chopped deli-style ham
- 10 ounces diced cooked chicken
- 1 cup peeled and diced potatoes
- ½ teaspoon dried thyme
- ½ teaspoon dried marjoram
- ½ teaspoon onion powder, or more to taste
- ¼ teaspoon garlic powder

- 1 (15.25 ounce) can whole kernel corn, undrained
- 1 (15 ounce) can cream-style corn
- 1 (10.75 ounce) can low-sodium chicken broth
- ½ cup low-fat (1%) milk

Directions

Step 1

Heat bacon drippings in 6-quart Dutch oven or stockpot over medium heat. Cook and stir ham in hot bacon drippings until slightly browned, about 5 minutes. Add chicken and potatoes to the pot; cook and stir until the potatoes soften slightly, about 5 minutes. Season the ham mixture with thyme, marjoram, onion powder, and garlic powder.

Step 2

Pour cans of whole kernel corn, cream-style corn, and chicken broth into the pot. Stir milk into the mixture. Bring the liquid to a boil, reduce heat to medium-low, and cook at a simmer until the potatoes are completely tender, about 10 minutes.

Cook's Notes:

You can use any type of cooking oil in place of the bacon drippings, but the bacon fat gives an extra layer of flavor.

Frozen hash brown-style potatoes can be used in place of the potatoes for even easier preparation.

Nutrition Facts

Per Serving: 290 calories; protein 20.6g; carbohydrates 34.8g; fat 9.2g; cholesterol 51.3mg; sodium 802.1mg.

Balsamic Marinated Chicken Breasts

Recipe Summary

Prep: 15 mins

Cook: 40 mins

Additional: 30 mins

Total: 1 hr 25 mins

Servings: 4

Yield: 4 chicken breasts

Ingredients

- ¾ cup balsamic vinegar
- ½ cup water

- 1 teaspoon dried minced onion
- ½ teaspoon crushed red pepper flakes
- ½ teaspoon dried minced garlic
- ¼ teaspoon salt
- ¼ teaspoon ground black pepper
- ¼ teaspoon paprika
- ¼ teaspoon crushed dried rosemary
- ¼ teaspoon dried parsley flakes
- ¼ teaspoon chili powder
- ⅛ teaspoon dried oregano
- 4 (6 ounce) skinless, boneless chicken breast halves

Directions

Step 1

Whisk together the balsamic vinegar, water, onion, red pepper flakes, garlic, salt, pepper, paprika, rosemary, parsley, chili powder, and oregano in a bowl, and pour into a resealable plastic bag. Add the chicken breasts, coat with the marinade, squeeze out excess air, and seal the bag. Marinate in the refrigerator 30 minutes to overnight.

Step 2

Preheat oven to 400 degrees F (200 degrees C). Line a baking sheet with aluminum foil, or lightly grease a broiler pan. Remove the chicken breasts from the marinade, and shake off excess. Discard the remaining marinade, and place the chicken breasts onto the baking sheet.

Step 3

Bake in the preheated oven until the chicken breasts are golden brown and no longer pink in the center, 30 to 40 minutes. An instant-read thermometer inserted into the center should reach 165 degrees F (74 degrees C).

Nutrition Facts

Per Serving: 222 calories; protein 35.7g; carbohydrates 8g; fat 4.3g; cholesterol 96.9mg; sodium 244.3mg.

Sugar-Free Whole Wheat Pumpkin Bran Muffins with Raisins

Recipe Summary

Prep: 15 mins

Cook: 25 mins

Total: 40 mins

Servings: 24

Yield: 24 muffins

Ingredients

- 2 cups raisins
- 2 cups whole wheat flour
- 2 cups wheat bran (such as Bob's Red Mill®)
- 2 tablespoons pumpkin pie spice
- 1 tablespoon baking soda
- 1 teaspoon baking powder
- 1 (29 ounce) can pumpkin puree (such as Libby's®)
- ¾ cup canola oil
- 4 eggs
- 1 tablespoon vanilla extract

Directions

Step 1

Preheat the oven to 350 degrees F (175 degrees C). Grease or line 24 muffin cups with paper liners.

Step 2

Plump raisins by microwaving them in a microwave-safe bowl with water to cover for 2 minutes. Drain water and set raisins aside.

Step 3

Combine flour, wheat bran, pumpkin pie spice, baking soda, and baking powder in a bowl.

Step 4

Combine pumpkin, canola oil, eggs, and vanilla extract in a separate bowl. Blend using an electric hand mixer on low speed. Add flour mixture and blend until combined. Fold in plumped raisins. Divide batter evenly between the prepared muffin cups.

Step 5

Bake in the preheated oven until a toothpick inserted into the center of a muffin comes out clean, about 20 minutes.

Nutrition Facts

Per Serving: 174 calories; protein 4g; carbohydrates 24.5g; fat 8.4g; cholesterol 31mg; sodium 262.8mg.

Whole Wheat Pumpkin Coffee Cake Muffins

Recipe Summary

Prep: 15 mins

Cook: 20 mins

Total: 35 mins

Servings: 12

Yield: 12 muffins

Ingredients

- Muffins:
- cooking spray
- 2 cups white whole wheat flour
- ½ cup brown sugar
- ¼ cup white sugar
- 2 teaspoons ground cinnamon
- 1 teaspoon baking soda
- 1 teaspoon salt
- ¾ cup pumpkin puree
- ¾ cup mashed ripe banana
- ½ cup vanilla Greek yogurt

- 2 tablespoons unsalted butter, softened
- 2 teaspoons unsalted butter, softened
- 2 large eggs
- 1 teaspoon vanilla extract
- Topping:
- 1 cup candied pecans
- ½ cup white sugar
- 2 teaspoons ground cinnamon

Directions

Step 1

Preheat the oven to 350 degrees F (175 degrees C). Spray a 12-cup muffin tin with cooking spray, or line with paper liners.

Step 2

Combine flour, brown sugar, white sugar, cinnamon, baking soda, and salt in a large bowl.

Step 3

Combine pumpkin puree, mashed banana, yogurt, butter, eggs, and vanilla extract in a large mixing bowl; beat with an electric mixer until well combined. Add dry ingredients and mix until just combined. Scoop batter into the prepared muffin cups.

Step 4

Mix pecans, sugar, and cinnamon together in a small bowl. Spoon or sprinkle on top of each muffin.

Step 5

Bake in the preheated oven until a knife inserted into the center comes out clean, 20 to 25 minutes.

Cook's Note:

You can use regular pecans or substitute walnuts for the candied pecans.

Nutrition Facts

Per Serving: 275 calories; protein 9.1g; carbohydrates 45.8g; fat 7.3g; cholesterol 38.6mg; sodium 416.6mg.

Homemade Wonderful Bread

Recipe Summary

Prep: 10 mins

Cook: 3 hrs

Additional: 15 mins

Total: 3 hrs 25 mins

Servings: 15

Yield: 2 pound loaf

Ingredients

- 2 ½ teaspoons active dry yeast
- ¼ cup warm water (110 degrees F/45 degrees C)
- 1 tablespoon white sugar
- 4 cups all-purpose flour
- ¼ cup dry potato flakes
- ¼ cup dry milk powder
- 2 teaspoons salt
- ¼ cup white sugar
- 2 tablespoons margarine
- 1 cup warm water (110 degrees F/45 degrees C)

Directions

Step 1

Whisk together the yeast, 1/4 cup warm water and sugar. Allow to sit for 15 minutes.

Step 2

Add ingredients in the order suggested by your manufacturer, including the yeast mixture. Select the basic and light crust setting.

Nutrition Facts

Per Serving: 162 calories; protein 4.5g; carbohydrates 31.6g; fat 1.8g; cholesterol 0.4mg; sodium 339.1mg.

Light Oat Bread

Recipe Summary

Prep: 5 mins

Cook: 3 hrs

Total: 3 hrs 5 mins

Servings: 12

Yield: 1 -1/2 pound loaf

Ingredients

- 1 ¼ cups water

- 2 tablespoons margarine
- 1 teaspoon salt
- 3 cups all-purpose flour
- ½ cup rolled oats
- 2 tablespoons brown sugar
- 1 ½ teaspoons active dry yeast

Directions

Step 1

Add ingredients to bread machine pan in order recommended by your manufacturer. Use regular light setting.

Nutrition Facts

Per Serving: 152 calories; protein 3.9g; carbohydrates 28.6g; fat 2.3g; sodium 216.2mg.

Marbled Chocolate-Pumpkin Muffins

Recipe Summary

Prep: 25 mins

Cook: 20 mins

Total: 45 mins

Servings: 12

Yield: 12 muffins

Ingredients

- 1 ¼ cups whole wheat flour
- 1 ½ teaspoons ground cinnamon
- 1 teaspoon baking powder
- 1 teaspoon baking soda
- ½ teaspoon ground cloves
- ½ teaspoon ground nutmeg
- ¼ teaspoon ground allspice
- ¼ teaspoon salt
- 1 cup pumpkin puree
- ½ cup pure maple syrup
- ½ cup plain whole-milk Greek yogurt
- 2 eggs, at room temperature
- ¼ cup unsalted butter, melted and cooled
- 2 teaspoons vanilla extract
- ⅓ cup dark cocoa powder (such as Hershey's® Special Dark), sifted
- ½ cup dark chocolate chips (Optional)

Directions

Step 1

Preheat the oven to 350 degrees F (175 degrees C). Grease a 12-cup muffin tin or line cups with paper liners.

Step 2

Whisk together whole wheat flour, cinnamon, baking powder, baking soda, cloves, nutmeg, allspice, and salt in a bowl until thoroughly combined.

Step 3

Whisk together pumpkin puree, maple syrup, yogurt, eggs, and melted butter in a second bowl until thoroughly combined and no lumps remain. Stir 1/2 of the flour mixture into the pumpkin mixture until just combined. Mix in the other 1/2 of the flour mixture and stir until just combined, making sure to not overmix.

Step 4

Divide batter evenly between 2 bowls. Whisk cocoa powder into one bowl until just combined. Fold chocolate chips into the other bowl. (Both batters will be somewhat thick.)

Step 5

Spoon about 1 tablespoon pumpkin batter and 1 tablespoon chocolate batter into each muffin cup. Continue filling muffin cups, alternating between both batters, until each cup is approximately 3/4 full. Make 2 or 3 swirls in the batter of each muffin with a bamboo skewer or butter knife, holding the muffin liner in place as you swirl. (The chocolate chips may make it difficult but just swirl around them.)

Step 6

Place muffins into the preheated oven and bake until a toothpick inserted into the center of the muffins comes out with a few moist crumbs, 19 to 23 minutes. Do not overbake.

Step 7

Cool in the tin for 5 minutes. Transfer to a wire rack to cool completely.

Cook's Note:

The combo of the batter being slightly thick, along with the use of chocolate chips, can make swirling the batter a bit tricky. Just make sure to hold the edges of the liners fairly securely and move the skewer/knife around as best you can. Don't swirl more than 2 or 3 times or it will lose its effect.

Nutrition Facts

Per Serving: 182 calories; protein 4g; carbohydrates 26.5g; fat 8.1g; cholesterol 43mg; sodium 263.9mg.

CONCLUSIONS

The Sjögren's syndrome diet reduces or eliminates foods that may trigger inflammation. Instead, it introduces foods rich in vitamins and minerals to create an anti-inflammatory effect. While it will not cure the disease, the Sjögren's syndrome diet may help treat symptoms such as dry mouth and dry eyes.

When combined with other treatment methods, it can provide a better quality of life and optimal health. With the inclusion of these healthy and delectable food choices as part of a Sjogren's syndrome diet, eating for optimum well-being is easy and pleasurable. Bon appetit!

The Sjögren's syndrome diet, similar to the anti-inflammatory diet, eliminates or reduces foods known to trigger inflammation. It instead introduces foods rich in vitamins and nutrients to create balanced meals. This diet is not a cure for Sjögren's syndrome, but it may help treat associated symptoms including dry mouth and dry eyes.

Combined with traditional treatment methods, the Sjögren's syndrome diet can help provide a higher quality of life and optimal health. Prior to pursuing this diet, discuss your expectations and options with your doctor to ensure you receive the best treatment.

www.ingramcontent.com/pod-product-compliance
Ingram Content Group UK Ltd.
Pitfield, Milton Keynes, MK11 3LW, UK
UKHW021655190726
13853UKWH00001B/269

9 798416 860943